NATURAL WAYS OF BOOSTING TESTOSTERONE

HOW TO BULK UP AND PUT YOUR SEX DRIVE IN OVERDRIVE

BY SMART READS

Visit:
www.smartreads.co/freebooks
to receive Smart Reads books for FREE

Check us out on Instagram:
www.instagram.com/smart_readers
@smart_readers

ABOUT SMARTREADS

Choose Smart Reads and get smart every time. Smart Reads sorts through all the best content and condenses the most helpful information into easily digestible chunks.

We design our books to be short, easy to read and highly informative. Leaving you with maximum understanding in the least amount of time.

Smart Reads aims to accelerate the spread of quality information so we've taken the copyright off everything we publish and donate our material directly to the public domain. You can read our uncopyright below.

We also believe in paying it forward and donate 5% of our net sales to Pencils of Promise to build schools, train teachers and support child education.

As a thank you for being a Smart Reader you can choose 3 FREE audiobooks from audible.com. Simply sign up for free by visiting www.audibletrial.com/Travis to get your first book.

After you sign up email me at Hello@SmartReads.co and tell me what other 2 books on audible you want and I will send you 2 Free Credits to download the books of your choice.

Thanks for choosing Smart Reads.

Sincerely,

Travis & the Smart Reads Team

TABLE OF CONTENTS

INTRODUCTION

Whenever testosterone is mentioned, most people conjure up thoughts of anger, aggression, and violence. However, this hormone has more to do with bodily functions, changes, and its vital role.

Nevertheless, there is a distinct impression given concerning the way testosterone affects a person's (both male and female) behavior in different situations. This hormone exists in males in quantities 8 times greater than in females, and it is what makes men display their unique masculine traits. Think of facial hair, development and growth of male reproductive organs, large sexual drive, the growth of bones and muscle, and even prevention of osteoporosis.

In other words, testosterone helps you stay healthy, and therefore we must ensure that the levels of this hormone do not drop. At the bottom part of the brain are two glands known as pituitary and cerebrum glands. These glands are responsible for the regulation of testes growth and testosterone is then secreted into the veins and arteries to play its vital role.

There are constant fluctuations in the levels of what is also known as the "t-hormone," with morning levels being higher than evening ones. There are times when testosterone tends to drop or stay within the lower levels. It is only in rare instances that we see the levels being excessively high. Whenever there is a lack of balance in the levels, a person can lose their health. You should always make a point to get your testosterone levels checked if you find yourself suffering any of the symptoms of low hormone levels.

Now that you have a basic understanding of what this hormone does and just how important it is, it is time to dive deeper into things. Both men and women are affected by this hormone, and you should not allow old age to convince you that it is normal for testosterone levels to reduce. Visit your physician regularly for checkups, get tested and seek professional advice.

CHAPTER 1: THE BIG T-HORMONE

We have so far clarified the significance of this hormone in the human body. Testosterone starts appearing when puberty hits, when facial hair starts appearing and muscles start popping out. It is a hormone present from conception. Without delving into the intricate details, let us examine how testosterone works in your body and what ways it is transported around.

Firstly, testosterone is produced in the male testes. Secondly, it is also a product of the androgen glands, though this is responsible for only a small amount of the hormone. However, both organ and glands are necessary for the production of testosterone, whose effects on the body are called "androgen effects."

During infancy, it is not easy to witness androgen effects. With time, the levels of testosterone increase, thus boosting the masculine characteristics within the brain. The effects of the hormone are not noticeable because the majority of the body parts aren't affected yet.

Then there is the pre-pubertal phase of testosterone where the external effects of the hormone are clearly evident to the person affected. Most people aren't fond of the side effects of this phase, which symbolizes the end of childhood. This is because it is normally characterized by acne, bad skin, and oily skin. Afterwards, there is the pubescent phase of life, which is a phase that everyone knows and most love. This means growth of facial hair above the upper lip, which most young men welcome. For women, this is not something that is viewed in the same light as men. Men also get sideburns, which were a great fashion statement back in the 1980s. Other effects also include pubic hair growth, development of body odor and maturation of the bones.

As testosterone is released during puberty, there are different body parts that are impacted in a number of ways. For example:

• Penile and clitoral enlargement
• Development of the Adam's Apple
• Development of muscles by men
• Growth and remodeling of the jaw-line
• Broadening of the ribcage and shoulders
• Deepening of the voice
• Full maturation of the bones

From all the information represented, you are now able to understand how this hormone controls different body functions and changes. Raising your testosterone levels is a direct way of enhancing your sex drive, as long as you can also adequately control these urges. Moreover, testosterone is also responsible for strengthening bones, muscles and intellectual aptitude.

Though testosterone treatment isn't the solution for everyone, it can definitely give you the boost you need when it comes to your sex drive. For women in their 20s, higher hormone levels are experienced compared to those in their 40s. For males, testosterone levels begin to drop when one crosses 30.

A reduction in t-hormone levels does not automatically mean lost sex drive, but it is possible. About 5% of the male population goes through the negative effects and reactions brought about by low testosterone levels, such as erectile dysfunction, weak erection, and loss of muscle and bone mass. About 10% of women suffer from low libido – in other words, low sex drive - due to low levels of testosterone.

CHAPTER 2: THE BENEFITS OF TESTOSTERONE

There are a lot of remarkable and wonderful benefits that testosterone provides to our bodies. We need to understand that this hormone goes way beyond just providing masculine features; it actually provides numerous health benefits. If a person suffers from low testosterone levels, then they will experience a number of ailments.

The first benefit of testosterone is fighting depression. Research has revealed that men who have low levels of this hormone tend to experience more signs of depression. In fact, the study showed that men who went for testosterone treatments were able to report an improvement in their moods and felt much better afterward. This should encourage you to go and get checked if you want to experience the magic of testosterone.

Apart from fighting depression, testosterone also has the ability to promote fat loss. It plays the role of maintaining your insulin and glucose levels, not to mention metabolizing fat. This means that any kind of reduction in T-hormone levels will lead to a disturbance in the levels and rate of the factors mentioned above. The ultimate outcome is an accumulation of fat and weight gain.

Accumulation of fat is terrible for your health and more so if you consider the fact that an increase in fat levels leads to a reduction in T-hormone levels. This is a vicious cycle where the initial cause later becomes part of the side effect. This entire theory also provides a straightforward explanation why men who are overweight tend to show greater estrogen levels and low T-hormone levels. The best way to break this cycle is to ensure that your testosterone levels are high, thus enabling you to live a life full of health.

The third benefit of testosterone in the body is the accumulation and growth of muscle tissue. Many different studies have concluded that the hormone helps build muscle. An increase in muscle mass results in an increase in strength, which is definitely a chick magnet. If you want to join a gym to bulk up, make sure that you get a physician to check out your T-hormone levels. You will be better off if you start getting treatment to boost your hormone levels.

When it comes to the human body, the heart plays a crucial role, thus it is important to make sure that it is well taken care of. Testosterone also helps in strengthening the heart and fighting diseases. An ongoing study has shown that testosterone actually protects against cardiovascular diseases by strengthening the cardiovascular system.

Your level of the T-hormone also affects bone strength. As men age, they become more susceptible to osteoporosis due to the drastic decrease in the levels of their testosterone hormone. This ultimately leads to weak bones and a combination of low testosterone and old age is not good. The reduction in testosterone hormone involves a process where the density of the bones reduces, thus limiting the ability of mineral absorption. The recommended solution is to see a doctor who will prescribe medication to boost your T-hormone levels.

Testosterone is the most critical hormone for sexual functioning and erections. If you find yourself suffering from any kind of sexual dysfunction or loss of sex drive, then the cause is pretty clear. In the event that there is a drop in libido or loss of interest in sex, go and get your testosterone levels checked.

Alzheimer's is a disease that afflicts the brain and gradually causes the rest of the body to deteriorate. It leads to memory and mobility loss, which can be scary for most people. The fact that it has no direct treatment makes things worse. However, research conducted by Hong Kong and South California Universities show that people with Alzheimer's have reduced levels of testosterone, thus revealing a connection between the T-hormone and brain functions. This also applies to memory loss and deterioration of brain tissue in elderly persons.

Testosterone is also a major factor in competitiveness, which plays a key role in maintaining the yearning to succeed. The hormone enhances your need to dominate and acquire power over others. It also helps in the seduction of the opposite sex and taking risks. This shows just how important it is for you to ensure that your T-hormone is at an optimal level.

CHAPTER 3: SYMPTOMS OF LOW TESTOSTERONE

What are the clear indicators of reduced testosterone levels in men? Once you determine that the hormone is not at the optimal level, how then do you figure out the cause?

There are some factors you have to consider. For example, have you had any recent injuries to your testicles? If so, tell your doctor this information so that they can consider it during treatment.

Another reason could be testicular cancer. There are many different cancers that are prevalent today, so make sure you go and get checked. In case you have already been diagnosed with cancer and have been undergoing treatment, you should also consider whether a change in medication is responsible.

Testosterone levels can also be affected by hormonal disorders, HIV/AIDS and any kind of infection. Always make sure that the medical facility you visit is sanitary. Aging is also a contributory factor, as well as chronic liver disease, obesity, Type 2 diabetes, and kidney disease.

The following are the indicators of a low testosterone level. They are sometimes erroneously regarded as due to aging, but you should carefully look into them when they arise.

• Erectile dysfunction and reduced libido – Testosterone functions as a sex hormone in both genders, so it is important to get yourself checked in case you suffer from low sex drive. In women, any changes in hormone levels generally result in mood swings.

• Increase in breast size – Testosterone is known to enhance the growth of muscle. If the levels drop, then there will be reduced muscle gain, which might affect the chest area. This leads to increase in the breast size in men.

• Reduced sperm count – If the quantity of semen becomes low during ejaculation, you need to get checked.

• Low bone density – Reduced bone mass is a clear indicator that something is wrong with your T-hormone levels.

• Hot flashes and mood changes.

• Hair loss – This usually infuriates most people, which is why many rush to buy hair products to spur growth. It is inevitable that there will be some hair loss as a person ages, but if you start losing body and facial hair then you may be deficient in testosterone.
• Tiredness and laziness – You begin to feel fatigued, lacking energy and sleepier than normal. If you used to exercise, you suddenly feel too tired to work out. You no longer run or lift heavy weights as strongly as you used to. This results in poor self-esteem and low

motivation. You may be getting enough sleep but you don't wake up feeling refreshed at all.

Hypogonadism
This condition is characterized by a reduction in testosterone due to the sex glands not producing enough or no sex hormones. This condition can be treated with medical care. Some of the symptoms of hypogonadism include:

In Males
- Damage to muscles
- Hot flashes
- Osteoporosis
- Erectile dysfunction
- Loss of hair
- Abnormal breast development
- Problems with concentration
- Tiredness
- Loss of libido
- Infertility
- Reduced growth of testicles and penis

In Females
- Elevated testosterone
- Lack of the feminine cycle
- Lack of libido
- Hot flashes
- Milky discharge from breasts
- Lack of breast development
- Little growth of hair on the body

It is important to note that an elevated level of testosterone is also dangerous. In men, it will result in excessive growth of facial hair, acne, and oily skin. In women, it results in infertility.

Therapy
The type of therapy that you get from a medical facility will depend on several factors. The first step is usually to take a blood test in order to determine the level of testosterone in the person's body. In case you have a low level, you may be advised to undergo treatment that may involve taking a generic hormone. This may be in the form of:

• A gel that is applied to the shoulders, upper arms, or stomach
• A patch placed on the scrotum or body two times daily
• A gum patch used two times every day

CHAPTER 4: FACTORS TO LOW TESTOSTERONE

Sleep
This is a critical factor in your testosterone levels. Failure to get adequate sleep will result in reduced T-hormone levels. In fact, research has shown that men who suffer from low testosterone experience fewer erections at night compared to men who have regular testosterone levels. To avoid this problem, you have to make sure that you get deep and adequate sleep without any disturbance. If this is difficult due to noise, then consider getting earplugs. If there is too much light, then get thicker curtains. Avoid staying up too late every night especially if you have to get up early to go to work.

Good Fats
Are you consuming the right kinds of fats? Is what you are eating benefiting your body? Will that food help you maintain your testosterone levels?

When you walk into a supermarket, you are likely to see food containing different types of fats. You should avoid picking any of them that contain a type of fat known as Trans Fats or partially hydrogenated oil. This type of fat is full of the bad kind of cholesterol and has been linked to atherosclerosis and heart disease. You should avoid products that contain this kind of fats, for example, cakes, and fast food.

Monounsaturated Fat

The following list contains foods that contain monounsaturated fats:

- Avocadoes
- Olive oil
- Poultry
- Nuts and nutty spreads
- Saturated fats

The Steps you Need to Take

Consume a dinner that contains a lot of monounsaturated fats and very little Trans Fats. If possible, eat an avocado with every dinner because it contains a high amount of monounsaturated fats. Eat eggs with the yolks, making sure that it is cooked with olive oil, macadamia or grass-fed margarine. Consume oily fish such as salmon a minimum of three times every week.

Take In More Nutrients

You need to consume three basic nutrients – Vitamin D, Zinc, and Magnesium. Researchers have discovered that people who start taking in Vitamin D show significant improvement in testosterone levels. You can get capsules from your local pharmacy or doctor. Vitamins are vital for a healthy life, so do not ignore them.

Zinc supplements can be used to boost testosterone levels in the blood of people who do not consume enough zinc. Severe and moderate zinc deficiency has also been linked to low T-hormone levels. It is clear to see that zinc supplements are a critical solution to low testosterone levels.

Another important mineral that serves numerous purposes in the body is magnesium. It is responsible for over 300 core biochemical bodily reactions. The process by which it does this is extremely complicated and cannot be explained here.

Magnesium is also known to stimulate rest and reduce fatigue (by blocking the anxiety hormone known as cortisol). Long periods of sound sleep and reduced levels of cortisol have both been linked to increased levels of testosterone. In conclusion, consuming more magnesium leads to better rest, lower cortisol and greater levels of testosterone. So what are the best sources of magnesium? Spinach and green leafy vegetables!

Exercise
If you find yourself living a sedentary lifestyle that does not incorporate much body movement, then your testosterone levels could be a problem. If you are male, exercise may be a solution.

Scientists and health experts are yet to conclude their research on exercise and its effect on testosterone, but one thing that is beyond doubt is that working out is important. Researchers at the California University discovered that testosterone levels went up 15 to 60 minutes after exercise. Though the results are still inconclusive, it is evident that there are many health benefits to exercising.

Men who suffer from reduced testosterone will not have any direct benefits just by exercising. It is not enough to have a significant impact. However, those men who suffer from extremely low testosterone levels will experience a significantly bigger impact.

CHAPTER 5: NATURAL WAYS OF RAISING TESTOSTERONE

In men, testosterone levels peak during young adulthood and begin to reduce by a small amount every year after that. The condition where the body fails to produce adequate amounts of testosterone is known as hypogonadism, or in some instances, "low T." There is testosterone treatment available to men who suffer from hypogonadism. However, this treatment is not used on men whose tests show that their testosterone levels are within the normal range for the person's age. Before we go into the topic of how you can raise your testosterone levels by natural means, let us take a look at some of the things that you should not do if you are intent on boosting your testosterone levels:

1. DON'T use testosterone supplements. Though you will end up feeling energetic after popping a couple of pills, and probably bulk up really quickly, they are not good for your health. They tend to be filled with caffeine, which may boost you temporarily but will cause harm in the long run. They also interfere with normal sleep and give you restless nights. For these reasons, they have been banned in some countries.

2. DON'T stay away from sunlight. Make sure that you get enough sunlight because it is one easy way of boosting your testosterone, not to mention prevent skin cancer. The ideal amount of Vitamin D is 800 to 1000 mg.

Tips for Naturally Boosting Testosterone
Your diet is a key component of naturally boosting
your testosterone level. Here are some of the ways
that you can naturally improve your testosterone
levels using the right diet:

1. Fish
Fish is a rich source of Vitamin D. It is good for the
heart, contains a lot of protein and has very few
calories. The fish can be the canned variety, but if you
can get fresh fish, then it would be better. One serving
is all that you need to hit your daily Vitamin D target.

In case fish isn't really one of your favorites, then you
can consider alternative sources of vitamin D. It is
important to remember to maintain some balance. A
diet consisting of too much Omega-3 fatty acids from
fish or other dietary sources could lead to an
increased risk of prostate cancer.

2. Milk
Milk is an extremely good source of vitamin D,
calcium, and protein. Women and children are advised
to take milk in order to build better bone health. Men
too can benefit from drinking milk in terms of bone
health as well as maintaining their testosterone level.
Always ensure that the milk that you buy has been
fortified with vitamin D. Just check the container and
read the label. Choose the skim or low-fat variety since
they offer you the same benefits that whole milk does
but without the excess fat.

3. Egg Yolk

Another extremely good source of vitamin D is egg yolks. Though egg yolk has a reputation for having high cholesterol, it is known to contain more health benefits compared to the egg whites. If you do not suffer from any cholesterol problems, then you can go ahead and enjoy one egg daily. If you have cholesterol issues, avoid egg yolks because too much cholesterol will reduce your testosterone levels.

4. Meat

There is a lot of concern over excessive consumption of meat. Not only does red meat contain more fat than chicken, but consuming too much of it has been linked to health conditions like colon disease. However, there are some meat varieties that can help boost your testosterone, for example, liver and ground hamburger. In order to restrict your consumption of animal fats to a limited level, choose lean cuts of burger meat and avoid consuming it excessively.

5. Sugar

Sugar is renowned for being a terrible ingredient that should not be consumed. Not only does it lead to a massive gain in weight, it also damages your ability to produce testosterone. Whenever you indulge in foods that are filled with sugar, be prepared for a sudden drop in testosterone.

Oranges contain a lot of vitamin C that is beneficial in boosting testosterone. Vitamin C has the ability to reduce your overall cortisol levels thus improving your testosterone levels. It is also critical for building a stronger and healthier skeleton, which then allows you to work harder during your exercise regimen. To get your dose of vitamin C, eat an orange every morning or you can also consider replacing the lettuce with spinach.

6. Chocolate

The regular male will rather eat a steak than a chocolate (though your average woman would not). However, it is beneficial to eat some chocolate once in a while. Chocolate is known to contain many biochemicals and agents that prevent cancer, boost your testosterone and provide several minerals and vitamins to the body.

However, there is one key precondition – the chocolate must be in its raw form. It is better to consume chocolate that contains a higher quantity of cocoa than a variety that only has a little cocoa.

7. Garlic

Garlic is a spice that acts as an additive for enhancing the taste of your food. Rather than using sugary or salty toppings and sauces to add flavor to your food, use garlic to spice up your food regularly with garlic. It is also known to help in the maintenance of testosterone levels. Regular consumption of garlic is known to boost health in several ways.

People who make it a habit to add garlic to their diet usually see an improvement in cardiac health as well as a rise in testosterone. It is recommended that you allow garlic to "sit" for a few minutes after you have peeled and chopped it, so as to enhance its health properties.

CHAPTER 6: TYPES OF SUPPLEMENTS TO BOOST TESTOSTERONE LEVELS

We have already seen just how critical testosterone is. It is the key male sex hormone though it is also important in the bodies of women. It helps in the building of muscle, loss of fat and improves optimal health.

However, there is a worrying trend in modern society that health experts have noticed. The testosterone levels of men are dropping at a very fast rate. In fact, men today are experiencing lower testosterone levels than ever before and this has been attributed to the unhealthy lifestyle society has embraced.

More and more men are finding it necessary to rely on testosterone supplements and boosters to increase their T-hormone levels. There are many different types of supplements being used and they work in either one of two ways:

• Some directly boost the testosterone hormone itself or other related hormones
• Some prevent testosterone from being turned into estrogen

Below is a list of testosterone supplements that will boost your hormone levels. These supplements are safe and have been scientifically verified through human trials.

1. D-Aspartic Acid

This is an amino acid that occurs naturally and is able to increase your low testosterone levels. Studies have shown that D-aspartic acid works primarily by raising the levels of your follicle-stimulating hormone as well as your luteinizing hormone.

Why is this important to know? The luteinizing hormone is the one that is responsible for triggering the Leydig cells, which are within the testes, to manufacture more testosterone. Scientists have conducted research in humans and animals and have discovered that a mere 12 days of taking D-aspartic acid is enough to raise luteinizing hormone levels. This also causes more testosterone to be produced and transported around the body.

D-aspartic acid has also shown an ability to enhance not only the production but the quality of sperms. Men suffering from low sperm production were given D-aspartic acid over a period of 90 days. At the end of the study, their sperm count had doubled.

In a separate study, athletic men who had great testosterone levels were put on a four-week weight-training regimen. Half of the men took 3 grams of D-aspartic acid every day. The results revealed that though both groups of men showed a significant increase in muscle mass and strength, the group that took the D-aspartic acid didn't experience any increase in testosterone.

So what is the bottom line? These studies reveal that D-aspartic acid is primarily beneficial to people who suffer from low testosterone or impaired sexual function. However, it may not make much of a difference if your T-hormone levels are already healthy. The recommended dosage is usually 2 to 3 grams for men who are deficient in testosterone.

2. Vitamin D

This is a fat-soluble vitamin that is produced whenever the skin is exposed to the sun's light. Within the body, it functions as an active steroid hormone. The reality is that in today's society, most people don't really get the sunlight exposure that they need. This eventually leads to most people becoming deficient in vitamin D.

One study discovered that increasing your vitamin D levels could boost testosterone and enhance the quality of sperm. It was also discovered that there is a close link between having a vitamin D deficiency and suffering from low testosterone. The participants of the study were asked to spend more time outdoors during summer and as their vitamin D levels rose, their testosterone levels did as well.

The bottom line is that vitamin D is vital for boosting your testosterone levels. You need to increase your exposure to sunlight, consume more foods rich in vitamin D, or take about 3,000 IU of vitamin D3 every day.

3. Tribulus Terrestris
This is an herb that is commonly used in herbal medicines and has been around for centuries. Tribulus has mostly been tested on animals and has proven to be effective in boosting the sex drive and raising testosterone levels.

Studies have also shown that men suffering from erectile dysfunction tend to experience an increase in sexual function and a 16% rise in testosterone levels. On the other hand, Tribulus does not seem to have an effect on men who have healthy levels of testosterone. The benefits of Tribulus are only experienced by men who have impaired sexual function and low T-hormone levels.

The bottom line is that Tribulus can help improve your sex drive, sexual function, quality of sperm, and testosterone levels.

4. Fenugreek
This is a very popular natural testosterone supplement. There is research that shows how fenugreek works in the human body, Fenugreek functions by lowering the enzymes that are responsible for converting testosterone into estrogen. A comprehensive 8-week study was conducted on two different groups of college students, each group consisting of 15 men. Every participant of the study undertook resistance training four times every week, with only one group of men being given 500 mg of fenugreek every day.

The group that received the supplement exhibited an increase in testosterone levels, not to mention an increase in strength and fat loss. However, the other group, which had not received the fenugreek, exhibited a slight drop in the hormone.

A second study was conducted to determine the effect of fenugreek on sexual performance and quality of life. Scientists took 60 healthy men aged 25 to 52 years old and split them into two groups. Group 1 was given a placebo pill daily for a period of six weeks. Group 2 was given 600 mg of fenugreek daily for the same 6-week period. The researchers discovered that the participants who had taken fenugreek reported an increase in strength, increased libido, enhanced sexual performance, higher energy levels, and better wellbeing.

The researchers concluded that a minimum of 500 mg of fenugreek supplement every day is enough to effectively boost testosterone and improve men's sexual function, regardless of whether they are healthy or deficient in the hormone.

5. Ginger
This is a spice that can be found in almost every household. It has been used for centuries as an alternative medicine, with research strongly suggesting that ginger lowers inflammation and increases testosterone levels.

The effect of ginger has been studied in rats with positive results. One study discovered that rats suffering from diabetes showed an increase in luteinizing and testosterone hormones after they were given ginger over a 30-day period. This increased the rat's sexual function. A separate study showed that ginger actually doubles the levels of testosterone in rats. A third study found that doubling the amount of ginger led to an even greater increase in testosterone.

One study was conducted in humans and involved 75 sterile men being given ginger supplements every day. After a three-month period, results showed that the men had a 17% rise in testosterone and a doubling of luteinizing hormone. There was also a 16% rise in sperm count.

The bottom line is that ginger is effective in increasing the sperm count and testosterone levels of men who are infertile.

6. Dehydroepiandrosterone (DHEA)

DHEA is a hormone that is found in the human body. It is responsible for regulating the level of estrogen and enhancing testosterone levels. Due to its effect on the body, it is a very popular way of improving testosterone.

Of all the supplements that can be used to boost testosterone, DHEA is the most extensively and well researched. Research has shown that that 50 mg to 100 mg of DHEA every day will boost testosterone by 20%. On the other hand, other studies have proved inconclusive when the same dosing amounts were used. Therefore, the results are somewhat mixed.

Due to the lack of clarity and agreement over the results of various studies, the effect of DHEA on testosterone is not conclusive. However, DHEA as a supplement is still considered a banned substance in professional sports.

In conclusion, DHEA is just like the other supplements and will help men with low testosterone levels. Though the research results are mixed, it is still popular as a booster and 100 mg a day is a safe and effective dose.

7. Zinc

Zinc is considered an aphrodisiac and is one of the essential minerals required by the body to perform over 100 chemical processes. Links have also been found between zinc and testosterone levels.

One study tried to measure the connection between zinc and testosterone. It discovered that reducing the intake of zinc led to a reduction in testosterone levels in healthy men. In fact, men who suffered from zinc deficiency reported an increase in testosterone levels after taking zinc supplements.

A second study measured how zinc affects infertile men who have normal or low levels of testosterone. The results showed that those men who suffered from low levels reported an increase in sperm count and testosterone. Those men who had normal hormone levels showed no extra benefit from the zinc supplement.

People who engage in stressful training routines, such as elite wrestlers, can prevent a drop in testosterone if zinc is taken every day. In other words, zinc supplements are beneficial for men who suffer from zinc deficiency and low testosterone, and elite athletes who find it difficult to recuperate from highly intense exercises.

8. Ashwagandha
This supplement is also referred to as Withania somnifera and is an Indian herbal medicine. Ashwagandha is mostly used as a medicine for relieving anxiety and stress.

The research was conducted on infertile men over a period of 3 months. They were given 5 grams of the supplement every day to test its effect on their sperm quality. The results showed a 10-22% rise in testosterone levels. Furthermore, the wives of 14% of the participants got pregnant.

Currently, it appears that ashwagandha improves testosterone levels and sexual function in men who are stressed, most likely by suppressing the stress hormone cortisol.

There are many different types of supplements out there that can be used to boost your testosterone levels. However, just a few of them have undergone any meaningful and conclusive research. These supplements have shown some benefits to people suffering from infertility and low testosterone.

Athletes and others who engage in strenuous exercise can also benefit from these supplements.

How to Triple Your Testosterone Levels

According to Tim Ferris, the author of The Four Hour Body, it is possible to triple your testosterone levels by adopting a specific diet. Ferris claims that he was able to drastically increase his testosterone by following a system consisting of four protocols. These four protocols are:

Protocol 1 – Long-term and sustained

• Brazil nuts – Take 3 nuts the moment you wake up and another 3 nuts before going to bed
• Vitamin D3 – Take 3000 to 5000 IU twice a day; when you wake up and before going to sleep.
• Fermented Cod Liver Oil and vitamin-rich butter fat - Take 2 pills in the morning and another 2 capsules at night.
• Brief cold showers or ice baths – Take a cold shower for 10 minutes in the morning and before going to bed

Let's get more specific with this particular diet. Brazil nuts are a great source of selenium. If your body is deficient in selenium then you should definitely be taking Brazil nuts.

According to Ferris, the optimum level of vitamin D3 in the blood is 55 nanograms per ml. Just make sure that you do not go over this limit and you will be OK. You can test your own vitamin D3 levels by using one of the many cheap test kits available.

For the fermented cod liver oil, you can take the Blue Ice brand that is made from a mixture of cod liver oil and butter fat. In case you cannot get the blend, then go for 1 capsule of cod liver oil and 1 capsule of butter fat. Use the dose explained above.

Lastly, there's the ice baths or cold showers. You may not enjoy these at first but you will quickly notice your health is improving.

Protocol 2 – Short-term
This involves boosting your testosterone within a 24-hour period. This protocol is great for prepping for a night out or having sex. The reason why you have to take these products before sleeping is because testosterone is produced from cholesterol, which is normally produced between 12 am and 6 am. It involves:

• 800 mg cholesterol at least three hours prior to going to bed, the night prior to having incredible sex
Make sure that 4 hours before having sex, take the following:
• 4 Brazil nuts
• 20 raw almonds
• 2 tablets Fermented Cod Liver Oil and butter fat

Protocol 3 – Increase protein intake
This helps you increase your testosterone levels, build muscle and burns fat. You will stay full the whole day. You should combine this step with extra strength training. You should choose whole food proteins (grass-fed meats) and high-quality whey. The

recommended amount is 1 gram per pound of lean body weight.

Protocol 4 – Get enough fats

Eat more fat of the saturated and polyunsaturated kind. The more good cholesterol you consume the greater you will perform in the sex department. The best sources of good fat include salmon and avocados.

Protocol 5 – Intermittent fasting

You should consider skipping breakfast on some days. This is because your testosterone levels tend to drop after you eat. You will also end up losing a bit of fat, which is great for your testosterone. The bottom line is that intermittent fasting maintains raging testosterone hormones.

CHAPTER 7: HOW TO USE TESTOSTERONE LIKE A PROFESSIONAL

Most people who already use or desire to use steroids to boost their performance in the gym will always opt for testosterone as the go-to supplement. This is because taking testosterone is one of the most effective ways of building muscle and strength quickly. If used properly, testosterone can help you become like one of those professional bodybuilders or MLB players. However, it is important to also note that testosterone use does come with side effects. The good news is that these effects can be avoided!

There are certain myths that must be addressed first before you learn how to use testosterone. The first one is that taking T-hormone supplements will give you "roid-rage." This is where someone is constantly violent beyond control. This is a big lie! It is true that some athletes tend to become overly aggressive due to the nature of their sport, but it is not the testosterone that made them this way. They were probably like that from the beginning.

The second myth is that testosterone supplements make your penis shrink. This is simply not true and may have been caused by people misunderstanding one of the side effects of misusing this hormone supplement. The fact is that testosterone may cause your testicles to shrink, but taking some simple steps, which will be discussed later on, can prevent this.

Safe Testosterone Usage

If you are a first timer, you can expect about a 40-pound gain in muscle within the initial three months. Once you stop using the steroids, you will lose some 15 pounds of water but still maintain the muscle. So where do you begin when you want to start taking testosterone supplements? Here are some tips:

1. Examine your goals

The first thing you need to do is determine if testosterone supplements are right for you. Examine your goals and find out if you want to lose fat or maybe gain muscle. If it is muscle growth and strength gain, then testosterone is OK, but if it's fat loss, then it is not the way to go.

2. Determine the form of testosterone to be used

You will have to decide which form of testosterone you want to use. There is no such thing as pure testosterone. It has to be combined with an ester in order to prevent the hormone flooding your system. The role of the ester is to enable the gradual release of the hormone in a timely manner.

You can go for testosterone Suspension (without an ester) which will enter your system in 1 day. There is testosterone Propionate which hits your system within 2-3 days. Testosterone Enanthate hits your system after 10 days. Then there is testosterone Sustanon, a combination of four different testosterones, which stays in your system for about 4 weeks. You should know that testosterone that acts very fast to enter your system tends to produce more side effects, in form of conversion to DHT and estrogen. What is recommended is that you choose the one that doesn't enter the system too fast but also choose one that doesn't take too long to act.

3. Find a reliable brand
There are numerous brands to choose from. Make sure you pick a brand that has great reviews and is reliable. There are some brands of testosterone supplements that are known to be cheap and unreliable. Some of these bad brands tend to cause negative side effects such as hair loss and acne. They may even be under-dosed and contain impurities. Go for potent brands like the Australian testosterone enanthate bladders.

4. The dosage and potential side effects
If you are a rookie who is just beginning to take testosterone, start with about 500 mg a week. Your supplement cycle should be something like this:

• Week 1 to week 10 – 500 mg testosterone enanthate every week
• Week 11 – 300 mg testosterone enanthate
• Week 12 – 200 mg testosterone enanthate

If you follow this cycle just as described above, you will definitely experience some nasty side effects, which are a result of the two paths that testosterone can take once it enters your system.

Testosterone can undergo either of two paths:
• 5alpha reductase can convert it into DHT

• It can be aromatized into estrogen

If it is converted into DHT, you may experience hair loss and an enlarged prostate. This may eventually lead to prostate cancer. To avoid these side effects, make sure that you take finasteride (also known as Propecia or Proscar). Finasteride is able to prevent the conversion of testosterone to DHT by 5alpha reductase. You can use the brand Fincar which is cheaper than Proscar but with the same effectiveness. Use 1.25 mg of finasteride daily per 500 mg of testosterone.

If testosterone is aromatized into estrogen, a condition called gynocomastia can develop in men. Gynocomastia is a side effect of steroids that is characterized by the permanent development of breasts. Though the breasts are small and harmless, it can cause a lot of embarrassment and mental trauma. The estrogen can also lead to fat gain, bloat, and water retention. On the other hand, eliminating this extra estrogen isn't difficult. You should consider taking an anti-aromatase such as Arimedex. This is the brand name for tablets that prevent the T-hormone from being turned into estrogen. Arimedex is sold in 1 mg tablets, so you should take about ¼ of a tablet every day for every 500 mg of testosterone you take. This drug has been proven to be safe.

One of the side effects of taking supplementation, and this one tends to scare most men, is the shrinking of the testicles. What happens is that the body detects an excess of testosterone and decides there is no need to produce anymore. This leads to shrunken testicles and a significant reduction in sperm count. You can avoid this by taking Clomid, which contains the chemical clomiphine citrate. It is recommended that you take 25 mg of Clomid daily for every 500 mg of testosterone you take. This substance stimulates the body to keep producing its own testosterone. The good news is that testicular shutdown is reversed once you stop taking steroids, and may take up to a month.

A second side effect of taking testosterone supplements is a rise in levels of cholesterol. You must have heard stories of people who suffer from heart attacks due to their steroid use. The problem isn't the steroids. It's the fact that they have continued consuming a diet filled with cholesterol while taking steroids. Get your blood tested and check your cholesterol as you begin your first cycle. If your cholesterol levels are already high, change your diet first.

Complete Beginner's Steroid Cycle

Week 1 – 10:
- 500 mg of testosterone every week
- 1.25 mg of Fincar daily
- 0.25 mg of Arimedex daily
- 50 mg of Clomid daily

Week 11:
- 300 mg of testosterone every week
- 1.25 mg of Fincar daily
- 0.25 mg of Arimedex daily

- 50 mg of Clomid daily

Week 12:
- 200 mg of testosterone every week
- 1.25 mg of Fincar daily
- 0.25 mg of Arimedex daily
- 50 mg of Clomid daily

Week 13:
- 1.25 mg Finasteride daily
- 0.25 mg Arimedex daily
- 100 mg Clomid daily

Week 14:
- 0.25 mg Arimedex after every 3 days
- 50 mg Clomid daily

If you have ever wanted to take testosterone and build muscle like a bodybuilder or MLB player, then this steroid cycle will help you start your journey. Most people tend to become confused about how to train or what to eat when taking testosterone supplements.

Firstly, since you will be building extra muscle, you will have to increase your daily calorie intake by about 2000 calories. Your protein intake should be increased by 2 grams for every pound of lean bodyweight. Your training doesn't have to change, but you can add 2 extra sets per week for every body part. Make sure that you get enough sleep, with the minimum being 8 hours every night.

Testosterone Injections

So far we have looked at taking testosterone supplements orally. However, in some special cases, testosterone is taken via an injection. Men and boys who suffer from impotence, hormonal imbalance or delayed puberty can be treated with testosterone injections. Women who suffer from breast cancer that is spreading all over their body are also treated using testosterone injections.

You should know by now that testosterone is not to be used for enhancing performance in sports. This book is about increasing your sexual drive and gaining muscle, so take every piece of advice here in the right context.

Men with prostate cancer, heart conditions, male breast cancer, kidney ailments, or severe liver disease should NOT receive testosterone injections. These injections must only be administered by a medical professional because misusing testosterone is dangerous.

Administration of the Injections

Testosterone is usually injected into the muscles. This is done at intervals of 2 – 4 weeks. The length of time that the treatment will be administered will depend on the condition you are suffering from. Throughout this period, it is important that you get regular blood work done. For boys who are receiving testosterone injections for delayed puberty, bone growth can be affected. Therefore, bone development should be checked using X-rays at intervals of 6 months. If you forget to go for a dose, just contact your physician for further instructions.

Side Effects

In case you experience any symptoms of allergies, go for emergency medical assistance. Some of the side effects of testosterone injections include hives; swellings on the throat, lips, face, and tongue; and difficulty breathing.

The presence of the following list of symptoms is cause for concern. For men, seek immediate medical advice if you experience:

• Nausea and vomiting
• Continuous penile erections
• Skin color changes
• Rapid weight gain
• Chest pain
• Swollen ankles
• Problems ejaculating
• Shrinking testicles
• Shortness of breath
• Painful urination
• Symptoms of blood clots in the lungs i.e. coughing blood, wheezing, chest pains.
• Symptoms of blood clots in the feet i.e. legs feeling warm, painful, and swollen
• Liver problems
• Excess calcium in the blood i.e. joint pain, constipation, confusion, tiredness, stomach pain

For women, contact your doctor immediately if you experience any of these symptoms:

• Hair growth like a man, for example, chest or chin hair
• Acne
• Enlarged clitoris
• Deepened voice
• Change in menstruation patterns

It is important to note that these lists of symptoms are not complete. Therefore, take the time to educate yourself further on the side effects of taking testosterone injections. Make sure that you are not taking any other drugs that may interact with the testosterone. If in doubt, ask your medical doctor.

CHAPTER 8: ANABOLIC STEROIDS – ARE THEY SAFE?

Anabolic steroids can be described as synthetic derivatives or variations of the sex hormone testosterone. The actual name given to this class of compounds is anabolic-androgenic steroids. The term "anabolic" simply means muscle building, while "androgenic" means having more masculine characteristics.

Back in the 1930s, it was discovered that anabolic steroids were able to boost muscle growth in test animals. These anabolic compounds were soon used to help treat devastating ailments in people.

After the 1950s, professional sportsmen and athletes began using anabolic steroids to boost their muscle strength and mass. Thereafter, scientists began making a wider variety of derivatives for use by athletes.

It is important to note that all steroids possess the same carbon structure. However, the different effects on the body are due to certain chemical alterations that have been made to the structure. Anabolic steroids are able to build muscle growth as well as induce the development of masculine sexual characteristics, such as facial hair and deep voice.

In some cases, doctors can prescribe anabolic steroids for people who are experiencing certain hormonal problems, for example, delayed puberty. They can also be used to treat conditions that usually lead to loss of muscle, for example, cancer and HIV/AIDS. However, anabolic steroids have been receiving a bad reputation because some people, primarily bodybuilders and athletes, have been abusing these drugs to enhance their sports performance or physical appearance. The question that needs to be answered is just how safe is the use of anabolic steroids? In order to do so, we must look at both sides of the coin. These drugs are safe and have their benefits when used the right way, for the right reasons, and administered by medical professionals. On the other hand, there are people who will abuse these drugs for their own selfish and personal reasons, and the negative side effects can be catastrophic. It all depends on how you choose to use anabolic steroids.

Abuse of anabolic steroids
Most of the people who abuse this form of steroids tend to do so either orally or via injections. The problem is that the doses that these people take tend to be 10 or sometimes even 100 times larger than what is normally recommended for patients. It is also possible to take anabolic steroids in the form of a patch, gel, or cream applied to the skin.

The people who tend to abuse these drugs often believe they can avoid the negative side effects or increase the positive effects by employing certain techniques. Some of these practices include:

- Cycling – This is where a person takes their doses over a specific period of time, stops for a while, and then resumes the dose.
- Stacking – This is where multiple different types of anabolic steroids are used together.
- Pyramiding – This is the practice of gradually increasing the dosage or frequency until you attain a peak, then slowly reducing (tapering) the dose back down.

The truth is that none of these three practices actually help you avoid the harmful side effects of anabolic steroids.

Anabolic steroids and your brain

Anabolic steroids do not function in the same way as other drugs that people abuse. They do not give you the same short-term impact on the brain as regular drugs do. Anabolic steroids will not make you high because they don't trigger the fast release of dopamine in the brain. However, they can still impact your neural pathways and chemicals, thus affecting your behavior and mood.

Short-term effects of steroid abuse

- Poor judgment
- Delusions
- Extreme irritability
- Extreme paranoia
- Severe acne

Long-term effects of steroid abuse

In men, the effects include:

- Liver damage
- Kidney failure
- High blood pressure
- Shrunken testicles
- Lowered sperm count
- Breast development
- Baldness
- Higher risk of prostate cancer

In women, the effects include:
- Liver damage
- Kidney failure
- High blood pressure
- Deepened voice
- Male-pattern baldness
- Growth of hair on the face and body

In teenagers, the effects include:
- Liver damage
- Kidney failure
- High blood pressure
- Stunted height
- Stunted bone growth

Addiction to steroids
It is possible for you to become addicted to anabolic steroids. Some continue to abuse these drugs even though they are causing physical harm, are expensive, and negatively affect relationships. Such behaviors are clear indicators of the potential of anabolic steroids to become addictive. Studies have also revealed that most steroid addicts end up turning to hard drugs, for

example, opioids, to relieve some of the negative side effects of the steroids. Some of the withdrawal symptoms of steroid abuse include:

• Reduction in sex drive
• Fatigue
• Mood swings
• Problems sleeping
• Cravings for steroids

Safe Steroid Use
Though it is true that anabolic steroids are controlled substances that pose a high risk of abuse and addiction, moderate and proper use of these drugs is possible. Just like any other drug or medication, the key lies in responsible use.

Firstly, it is important to know the medical conditions that you have before you start taking anabolic steroids. If you have intolerance to them or have some kind of inherent medical problem, do not take these drugs.

The following medical conditions disqualify a person from using steroids unless your doctor has prescribed them:

• Liver disease
• Kidney disease
• Diabetes
• Coronary artery disease
• Heart disease
• High blood pressure

• Alcoholism

Using the right dosage and cycle length
Anabolic steroids, when used in the proper doses and for the right cycle lengths, can be beneficial. The biggest mistake that most abusers make is that they take too much or they take the steroids for too long. If you want to gain muscle, you need to realize that there is a lot of hard work involved. You must spend time finding the right dose for your own personal performance. You must ensure that you know how to time the cycles so that you avoid the harmful side effects. All this requires comprehensive research on your part since different products have different doses and cycle lengths.

Collecting the right supplements and PCT substances
As long as you use the necessary supplements and undertake post-cycle therapy (PCT) after your cycles, you will be fine. Doing this will prevent you from suffering the negative side effects. There are certain supplements that you need to have as you take your anabolic steroids:

• Testosterone – Taking anabolic steroids blocks the natural production of testosterone. This means that you must take testosterone in an exogenous form. Just make sure you take them in the proper amounts.
• Aromatase inhibitors – Such compounds block the body from producing aromatase, the enzyme that turns anabolic steroids and excess testosterone into estrogen.

• Omega-3 fatty acids – It has been shown that steroids can cause a rise in bad cholesterol levels and reduction in good cholesterol. These fatty acids can prevent this to some level.

• Milk thistle – as a natural plant-based compound, milk thistle protects your liver from damage caused by the steroids.

PCT is dependent on the type of steroids you are using and how long you have been using them. These are some of the PCT supplements you may require:

• SERMs (Selective Estrogen Receptor Modulators) – SERMs are designed to block estrogen, stimulate the production of follicle stimulating hormone (FSH), and luteinizing hormone (LH). These hormones will normalize your testosterone levels.

• HGH (Human Growth Hormone) – You should start using this compound around 4 weeks prior to the end of the cycle. Keep using it for 12 weeks after the end of the cycle.

In spite of the social stigma over the use of anabolic steroids, you can safely use these products in conjunction with the appropriate supplements, diet and exercise regimen.

CONCLUSION

When all is said and done, you have to take your health seriously. You have to make the commitment to eat healthy foods every time so that you are in optimal health. You also need to adopt a lifestyle that includes enough exercise to keep you active. Of course, this will be easier if you can find an exercise partner who will be willing to assist you with your regimen. Make sure that your workouts push you to your limits so that you can reap the maximum benefits. Just like all the other parts of your body, your testosterone hormone plays a crucial role and must be kept at the right optimum level. Remember – too much of something is also dangerous to your health.

You need to understand that testosterone as a hormone is what makes a man who he is. Testosterone is produced naturally by the body and is responsible for numerous vital functions within the body of the male species. Some of these functions include the building of muscle, self-confidence, aggression, motivation, and much more.

Most of the characteristics that make a person distinctively male are expressly due to their level of testosterone. For example, men tend to be described as having a dominating, alpha-male attitude. A man's high motivation levels are also linked to his testosterone hormone.

Apart from just causing the building of lean muscle, testosterone is also responsible for maintaining a trim waistline. Maintaining the right levels of the testosterone hormone will help you avoid developing the extra layers of fat that tend to accumulate around the abdomen, especially in men who are aging. It is the testosterone that enables a person to develop a six-pack when they exercise.

It is important to note that loss of hair from your head or a decrease in sexual drive should not be attributed to the normal aging process. Testosterone plays a key role in every stage of life, all the way from giving you a deep voice, growing your facial hair, and causing your sexual organs to grow larger. Whenever you feel that you are unusually tired, depressed, and are experiencing a loss of sexual strive, you need to visit a medical facility to get your testosterone levels checked out.

Though ailments like depression, hypertension, heart disease, and diabetes are not usually associated with having low testosterone levels, research conducted years ago proved that there is a link between these two sets of conditions. If you are experiencing any of the above diseases, then it is recommended that you also ask your doctor to test your T-hormone levels.

Every man knows just how important testosterone is to their manhood and their health. It is sad that most men fail to understand its impact. The reality is that as a man grows older, his testosterone levels will naturally drop, but there are ways to prevent this from happening. That is what this book is essentially about.

We hope you have learned as much about testosterone as you can. Please feel free to go through this book as often as necessary to make sure that you take the appropriate measures to maintain your testosterone to bulk up and get your sex drive back!

THANKS FOR READING

We really hope you enjoyed this book. If you found this material helpful feel free to share it with a friend. You can also help others find it by leaving a positive review where you purchased the book.

The Smart Reads library is growing by the day! Make sure and check out the other wonderful books we have in our catalog and let us know which ones are your favorite.

Visit:
www.smartreads.co/freebooks
to receive Smart Reads books for FREE

Check us out on Instagram:
www.instagram.com/smart_readers
@smart_readers

Don't forget your 3 FREE audiobooks. Use this link www.audibletrial.com/Travis to signup for a FREE audible account and then email me at Hello@SmartReads.co and let me know which other two books you want and I will send you credits to download the books for free!

WHY I STARTED SMART READS

I started smart reads because every time I want to learn about something new I'd have to buy 20 books on the topic and spend way too long sorting through them and reading them all until I can arrive at the big picture. Until I had enough perspectives to know who was just guessing, who was uninformed and who had stumbled upon something remarkable.

I wished someone else could just go in and figure that out for me and tell me what matters. That's how Smart Reads was born. I want Smart Reads to be a company that does all that research up front. Sorts through all the content that is available on each topic and pulls out the most up to date complete understanding. Then have people smarter than me package the best wisdom in an easy to understand way in the least amount of words possible.

For example, I got a new puppy so I wanted to learn about dog training. I bought 14 different books about dog training and by the time I got through the first 5 and finally started seeing the big picture on the best way to train my puppy, she had grown up into a dog.

Yeah she's well behaved. She doesn't poop in the house. I can get her to sit and come when I call. But what if someone else went in and read all those books for me. Found the underlying themes and picked out the best information that would give me the big picture and get me right to the point. And I'd only have to read one book instead of 15. That would be amazing. I would save time. And maybe my dog would be rolling over, cleaning up after my kid and doing the dishes by now.

That my friends, is the reason I started smart reads. Because I wanted a company I can trust to deliver me the best information in an easy to understand way that I can digest quickly. Because dog training is one of many subjects I want to master and bring into the rest of my life. And the quicker I can learn a wide variety of topics the sooner that information can begin playing a role in shaping my future. And none of us knows how long that future will be. So why not do everything we can to make the best of it.

WE WANT TO HELP PLANT A BILLION TREES

For every 10 hardcover books we sell we are going to plant a tree in collaboration with www.plantabillion.org to make up for the paper we use printing the books and to do our part helping to regain our valuable forests.

SMART READS ORIGINS

Smart Reads was born out of the desire to find the best information fast without having to wade through the sheer volume of fluff available for purchase. Smart Reads combs through massive amounts of knowledge accessible online and compiles all the best into easily digestible books on a wide variety of subjects.

We consider ourselves Smart Readers, not dummies. We like to learn a TON about a WIDE variety of topics. It's the best way to capture the big picture! With the amount of noise in the marketplace today, each new topic we try to learn about begins with a never ending search to find facts that matter. It becomes a treasure hunt rather than an education.

Smart Reads aims to be your one-stop-shop for superior information on any subject you want to learn about. When you see a Smart Reads book on your topic of interest you know your search for quality information is over. As a smart reader, you get more information on more topics in less time.

OUR MISSION

Smart Reads mission is to accelerate the spread and availability of valuable information. We believe having access to knowledge is a basic human right and want to see every person on the planet be able to learn about any topic that would enhance their lives. We hope to remove barriers to sharing by taking the copyright off everything we publish and donating it to the public domain.

We also know we can't accomplish this mission by ourselves so we are giving 5% of our net profit to Pencils of Promise. We hope to donate $1,000,000 or more by 2020 to build over 2,000 schools and increase educational opportunities in the developing world.

By purchasing from Smart Reads you are contributing to helping kids all over the globe get access to a valuable education they otherwise wouldn't have had.

Doesn't it feel good knowing that by educating yourself you are helping to educate the next generation!? We think so too...

Thanks for choosing Smart Reads! You Smart Reader you...

Travis and the Smart Reads Team

Customers Who Bought This Book Also Bought

Success Principles: Techniques for Positive Thinking, Self-Love and Developing a Powerful Mindset

Probiotic Dieting: The Miracle of Probiotics in Healing Your Gut, Trimming Belly Fat and Weight Loss

Kundalini Awakening: Techniques To Raise Your Shakti Energy

How To Control Alcoholism: Proven Techniques to Stop Alcohol Abuse, Overcome Dependency, Break Addiction and Recover Your Life

Develop Self-Discipline: Daily Habit to Make Self Confidence and Will Power Automatic

Meditation Magic: Free Yourself from Worry, Depression, Stress and Anxiety

How To Run: Beginner Running Program. Learn to Run. Running to lose weight. Runner Form. Fun Run.

Self-Esteem Supercharger: Build Self Worth and Find Your Inner Confidence

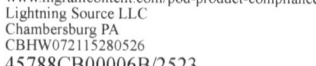